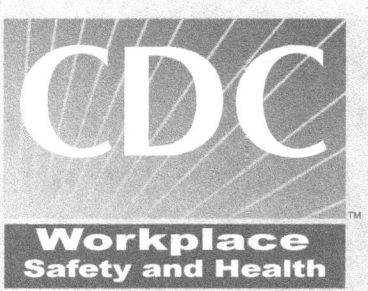

# Environmental Assessment for the Presence of Influenza Viruses (2009 Pandemic Influenza A H1N1 and Seasonal) in Dental Practices – Ohio

*Steven H. Ahrenholz, PhD, MS, CIH*
*Scott E. Brueck, MS, CIH*
*Marie A. de Perio, MD*
*Francoise Blachere, MS*
*William G. Lindsley, PhD*

Health Hazard Evaluation Report
HETA 2010-0019 & 2010-0021-3120
January 2011

DEPARTMENT OF HEALTH AND HUMAN SERVICES
Centers for Disease Control and Prevention

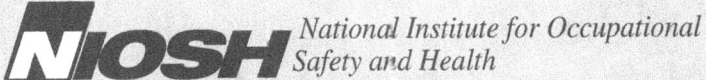 National Institute for Occupational Safety and Health

The employer shall post a copy of this report for a period of 30 calendar days at or near the workplace(s) of affected employees. The employer shall take steps to insure that the posted determinations are not altered, defaced, or covered by other material during such period. [37 FR 23640, November 7, 1972, as amended at 45 FR 2653, January 14, 1980].

# CONTENTS

# ABBREVIATIONS

| | |
|---|---|
| °C | Degrees Celsius |
| °F | Degrees Fahrenheit |
| µl | Microliter |
| µm | Micrometer |
| µM | Micromole |
| ACGIH® | American Conference of Governmental Industrial Hygienists |
| ACIP | Advisory Committee on Immunization Practices |
| CDC | Centers for Disease Control and Prevention |
| cm2 | Centimeters squared |
| cDNA | Complimentary deoxyribonucleic acid (DNA) |
| GSD | Geometric standard deviation |
| HELD | Health Effects Laboratory Division |
| HHE | Health hazard evaluation |
| HHPC | Hand Held Particle Counter (ART Instruments, Inc., Grants Pass, Oregon) |
| ILI | Influenza-like illness |
| ID | Internal diameter |
| ISO | International Organization for Standardization |
| Lpm | Liters per minute |
| mL | Milliliter |
| mm | Millimeter |
| NA | Not applicable |
| NAICS | North American Industry Classification System |
| NIOSH | National Institute for Occupational Safety and Health |
| NP | Nasopharyngeal |
| pH1N1 | 2009 pandemic influenza A (H1N1) |
| PPE | Personal protective equipment |
| PTFE | Polytetrafluoroethylene |
| qPCR | Quantitative polymerase chain reaction |
| RNA | Ribonucleic acid |
| RSV | Respiratory syncytial virus |
| RT-PCR | Reverse transcription polymerase chain reaction |
| SHEA | Society for Healthcare Epidemiology of America |
| T1 | First stage centrifuge tube of bioaerosol sampler |
| T2 | Second stage centrifuge tube of bioaerosol sampler |
| WHO | World Health Organization |

# HIGHLIGHTS OF THE NIOSH HEALTH HAZARD EVALUATION

**The National Institute for Occupational Safety and Health (NIOSH) received requests for health hazard evaluations from two dental practices (one general and one pediatric) in a metropolitan area of Ohio. Management at each dental practice was concerned about transmission of 2009 pandemic influenza (also known as flu) A (H1N1) (pH1N1) virus to dental staff.**

## What NIOSH Did

- We visited each dental practice four times over a 6-week period beginning in late January 2010.
- We collected air and surface samples in both dental practices on eight separate dates.
- We collected nasopharyngeal samples from dental staff.
- We tested all samples for pH1N1 and seasonal flu viruses.
- We administered a flu symptom survey to dental staff.
- We reviewed information about flu symptoms among patients.

## What NIOSH Found

- No pH1N1 virus was found in the air or surface samples at either dental practice.
- Seasonal flu virus was found in the air at the pediatric dentistry practice during one visit.
- Dental staff did not come to work while ill.
- Vaccination rates for both seasonal and pH1N1 were low for staff at both dental practices.

## What Managers Can Do

- Encourage employees to get the seasonal flu vaccine every year.
- Develop procedures for tracking ill employees and excluding them from work.
- Screen patients for flu symptoms before their visits or at the time of check-in.

## What Employees Can Do

- Get the seasonal flu vaccine every year.
- Self assess for flu symptoms.
- Report any symptoms to management as soon as possible.
- Do not report for work when ill.

*This page intentionally left blank.*

# SUMMARY

No 2009 pandemic influenza A H1N1 virus was found in any air or surface samples at two dental practices, but seasonal influenza A was found in the air of the pediatric dental practice. Influenza vaccination rates for staff at the dental practices were below national rates for healthcare personnel during the 2009–2010 influenza season. We recommend that all staff get the seasonal influenza vaccine every year.

In October 2009, NIOSH received requests for HHEs from the management of two dental practices in a metropolitan area of Ohio. The dental practices were concerned about transmission of pH1N1 to dental employees. NIOSH investigators visited each dental practice four separate times over a 6-week period beginning in January 2010. During each site visit, we collected air and surface samples for pH1N1 and seasonal influenza virus. Air samples were collected with bioaerosol samplers that separated airborne particles into three size ranges: $\geq 4.1$ µm; 1.0–4.1 µm; and $\leq 1.0$ µm aerodynamic diameter. Air samples were collected near patients in exam chairs and at a distance of several feet from patients to distinguish between large and small airborne influenza particles. We also collected NP swabs from dental staff, administered a influenza symptom survey to dental staff, and reviewed symptom surveys that the dental practices had asked patients to complete.

No pH1N1 or seasonal influenza A virus was detected in the 48 air samples or 52 surface swab samples we obtained at Dental Practice A, a general dentistry practice. No pH1N1 virus was detected in the 48 air samples collected at Dental Practice B, a pediatric dentistry practice. However, we identified a seasonal influenza A strain (H3N2) ($\leq 1$µm in size) from air samples collected near patient exam chairs in three exam rooms at Dental Practice B on March 2, 2010. No pH1N1 or seasonal influenza A virus was found in the 54 surface swabs collected in Dental Practice B.

All NP samples collected from dental practice staff at both practices were negative for influenza A viruses. During our sampling dates, none of the dental staff who completed the influenza symptom survey at Dental Practice A had ILI in the prior 7 days. Only one dental staff member who completed the survey at Dental Practice B had ILI in the prior 7 days. Of those who completed the survey at Dental Practice A, only two patients or individuals accompanying patients had ILI in the prior 7 days. At Dental Practice B, six patients or individuals accompanying patients had ILI in the prior 7 days. For staff at Dental Office A, 8% reported getting the pH1N1 vaccine and 25% reported getting the seasonal influenza vaccine. Of the staff at Dental Practice B, 18% reported getting both the pH1N1 and seasonal influenza vaccine.

Exposure of dental staff at both practices to airborne pH1N1 and seasonal influenza A viruses during the sampling days appears to have been limited. This may be because the community influenza incidence during the time of our evaluation was below typical seasonal influenza levels. The absence of positive surface swab samples for pH1N1 or seasonal influenza may be primarily due to the low number of patients reporting ILI.

We recommend that all employees get the seasonal influenza vaccine every year. Employees should self-assess for influenza symptoms and not report to work if ill. Dental practices should monitor and manage employees who are ill and absent. Additionally, dental practices should consider developing mechanisms to screen patients for ILI symptoms prior to their visits or at the time of check-in. Dental practices should advise patients to consider postponing visits and procedures that are not urgent until 24 hours after the patient is free of fever, especially in times of high influenza activity within the community.

**Keywords:** NAICS 621210 (Offices of Dentists), dental practice, dentist, seasonal influenza, H1N1, pandemic influenza, swine flu, bioaerosol

# INTRODUCTION

We received requests for HHEs from the management of two dental practices in a metropolitan area of Ohio. The management at both dental practices was concerned about transmission of pH1N1 virus to dental employees.

Because the methods and issues were the same for both dental practices, the investigations are discussed together in this report. Our primary objective for these evaluations was to assess dental practice employees' potential for exposure to pH1N1 and seasonal influenza viruses at work. The questions we sought to answer were:

- Are pH1N1 or seasonal influenza viruses present in the workplace?

- Are workers potentially exposed to airborne pH1N1 or seasonal influenza viruses (size range < 4.1 μm aerodynamic diameter) in their breathing zone or in the immediate proximity of patients (approximately 3 feet or less)?

- Are influenza viruses, if present within the workplace, capable of being collected as an airborne particulate < 4.1 μm aerodynamic diameter at distances beyond the immediate proximity of the source (greater than 3 feet)? (Note that the maximum distance at which droplet transmission may end and the minimum distance at which airborne transmission is considered to occur remains unresolved [Siegel et al. 2007]).

The methods available to us at the time of this evaluation allowed for the identification of influenza viruses in the work environment but could not determine if these viruses were viable and capable of causing illness. Presence of the influenza virus does not by itself indicate risk of infection. Additionally, the amount of virus found cannot be used by itself to assess the likelihood of infection or illness. However, if viruses are detected, this indicates the potential for exposure.

The focus of this evaluation was to determine if pH1N1 and/or seasonal influenza viruses are present in a workplace such as a dental practice, which does not perform aerosol generating healthcare procedures. Aerosol generating procedures are considered to increase the risk of influenza transmission to employees. Dental practice employees are unlikely to encounter individuals seeking care for influenza symptoms or complications, although these individuals may visit the dental practice despite having influenza symptoms.

## Background on the Dental Practices

Dental practice A provides general dentistry services to adults and children over the age of three. The majority of patients are adults. The practice employs two dentists, four dental hygienists, three dental assistants, and two administrative staff. Dental practice B provides pediatric dentistry services for children ages 1 to 18 years of age. A majority of patients are in the 1 to 10 year age range. This practice employs two dentists, three dental hygienists, six dental assistants, and three administrative staff.

## Background on 2009 Pandemic Influenza A (H1N1) Virus

The pH1N1 virus, also referred to initially as "swine flu," was first detected in humans in the United States in April 2009. On June 11, 2009, the WHO signaled that a pandemic of pH1N1 was underway. CDC estimated that, between April 2009 and April 2010, 43–89 million cases of pH1N1, 195,000–403,000 pH1N1-related hospitalizations, and 8,870–18,300 pH1N1-related deaths occurred [CDC 2010a].

Spread of the pH1N1 virus is thought to occur in the same way that seasonal influenza spreads [CDC 2009a]. Influenza viruses are spread mainly through droplet transmission though evidence for airborne transmission and transmission via direct contact also exists [CDC 2009a].

The symptoms of pH1N1 infection include fever, cough, sore throat, runny or stuffy nose, body aches, headache, chills, and fatigue. Some patients have had vomiting and diarrhea, while some patients have respiratory symptoms without a fever. Illness with the pH1N1 virus has ranged from mild to severe. While most people who have been sick have recovered without needing medical treatment, hospitalizations and deaths from infection with this virus have occurred. Many people who have been hospitalized with this pH1N1 virus have had one or more medical conditions previously recognized as placing people at "high risk" of serious seasonal influenza-related complications, including pregnancy, diabetes, heart disease, asthma, and kidney disease [CDC 2009a].

## Background on Influenza Vaccines

The pH1N1 vaccine became available in the United States in October 2009. In July 2009, CDC's ACIP recommended that certain groups of the population receive the pH1N1 vaccine first [CDC 2009b]. These target groups included all healthcare personnel, including employees in outpatient clinics such as dental care settings. In July 2009, CDC's ACIP updated its longstanding recommendations for seasonal influenza vaccination [CDC 2009c]. The groups targeted for this vaccine were similar to those for the 2009 pH1N1 vaccine and also included all healthcare personnel, including employees in outpatient clinics such as dental care settings.

The assessment methods are described in general below. Additional details are found in the appendix to this report.

## Environmental Assessment

We visited each dental practice on 4 days over a period of 6 weeks beginning in January 2010. Each week we asked both practices to identify their busiest days for the upcoming week. We selected the days for our evaluation that involved greater patient scheduling and the presence of most of the dental practices' staff.

We collected aerosols with a two-stage cyclone bioaerosol sampler (Figure 1) developed and used by other NIOSH investigators to identify the presence and size fraction of airborne pH1N1 and seasonal influenza viruses and viral fragments [Lindsley et al. 2006; Blachere et al. 2009]. The bioaerosol samplers allowed for the collection of pH1N1 and seasonal influenza virus and viral particles across three size fractions: $\geq 4.1$ μm; $1.0-4.1$ μm; and $< 1.0$ μm aerodynamic diameter.

We collected air samples in five patient rooms and the receptionist area over 4 days between January 27, 2010, and February 24, 2010, at Dental Practice A. At Dental Practice B, we collected air samples in six patient rooms and the reception desk area on 4 days between January 26, 2010 and March 2, 2010. We collected environmental samples at each practice 1 day per week and limited sampling duration to between 4 and 5 hours because of concerns about excessive desiccation of viruses during longer sample periods. Samples were collected during the first half of the workday on the days considered by the practices to be their busiest. RT-PCR analyses were used to identify the presence of pH1N1 and seasonal influenza virus and viral particles collected by the air samplers. RT-PCR analyses for the presence of RSV were added for the last 3 days of environmental sampling at Dental Practice B. RSV is a common respiratory illness that occurs in children and has been evaluated previously along with air sampling for influenza virus [Lindsley et al. 2010].

The bioaerosol samplers were mounted in two locations within patient rooms. One was positioned about 2 to 3 feet from the potential source (patient) of pH1N1 or seasonal influenza virus, depending upon where the dental staff positioned the exam light while they were working, and was usually located on the dental exam light support structure (Figure 2). This placed the sampler within approximately 3 feet of dental staffs' breathing zone when they did exams and procedures. Dental staff positioned the exam light closer while working with a patient and pushed it up and away when finished. The objective of using this spacing was to determine if we could find influenza virus in the area where droplet and large aerosol transmission is thought to occur (within approximately 3 feet) [Siegel et al. 2007].

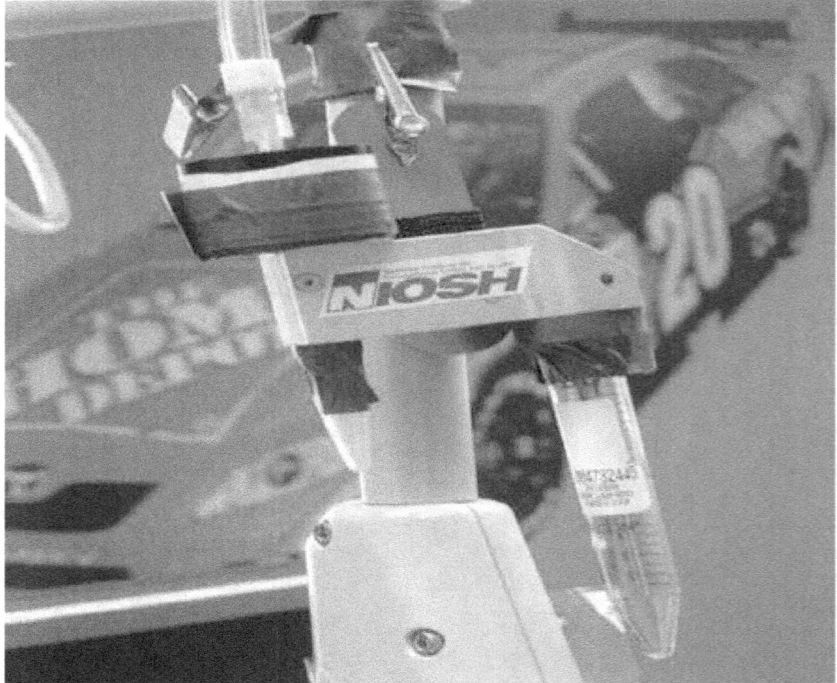

Figure 1. Close-up of NIOSH two-stage cyclone bioaerosol sampler mounted on dental light fixture.

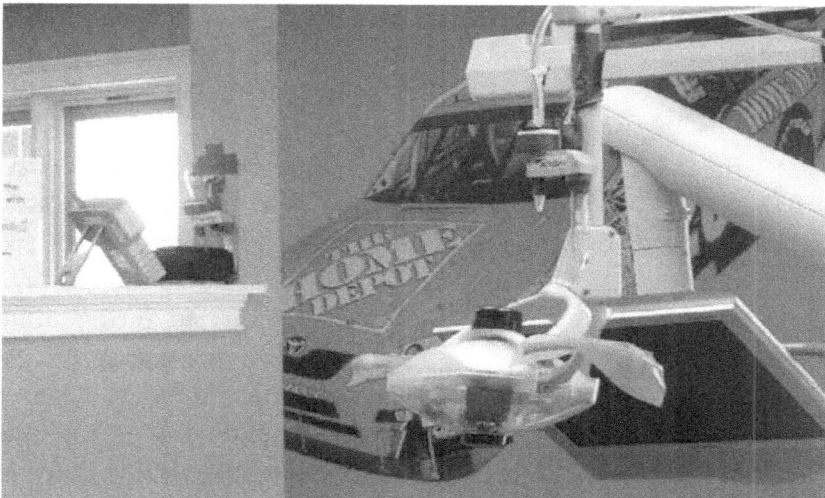

Figure 2. Two-stage NIOSH cyclone bioaerosol sampler attached to support above dental exam light at Dental Practice B.

A second sampler was located approximately 4 to 8 feet (Dental Practice A: average 6.6 feet; Dental Practice B: average 5.9 feet) from the potential source. This distance would allow us to assess whether influenza virus spreads farther than the immediate 3-foot vicinity of the source. Influenza virus collected by the distant sampler would more likely be present in small (< 4.1 μm) airborne particulates that remain suspended within the room and carried beyond the region where droplet transmission typically occurs. Depending on the room configuration, we placed the second sampler on a tripod in the corner of the room, on a short wall between rooms, on top of a small wall cabinet, or on an elevated location above and behind the patient exam chair (Figure 3). The size of the patient rooms and configuration of equipment was such that maintaining minimum distances for our second samplers of at least 6 feet was not always possible.

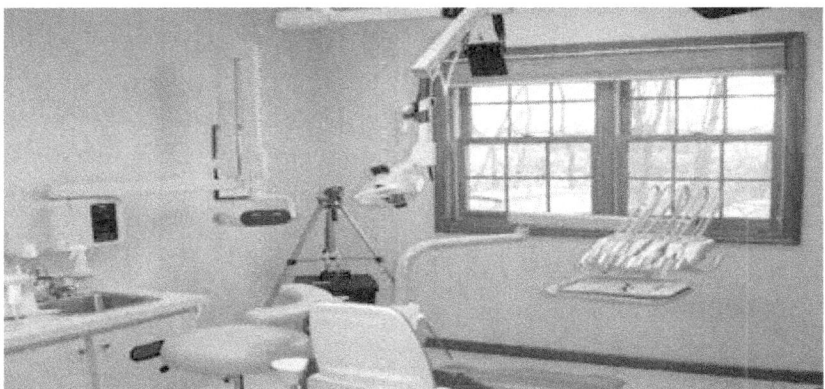

Figure 3. Two-stage bioaerosol sampler mounted on a tripod in the corner of an exam room at Dental Practice A. (Note: Additional sampler on support arm of exam light above dental chair.)

We collected surface swab samples (swabs – Copan Diagnostics, Corona, California; phosphate buffer to moisten swabs – Invitrogen, Aukland, New Zealand) in each room where we took air samples to evaluate whether pH1N1 or seasonal influenza virus was present on surfaces in close proximity to patients and on work surfaces used by the dental staff. Other investigators have previously identified the presence of influenza A virus on up to 50% of household and daycare center fomites and classroom surfaces tested during influenza season [Boone and Gerba 2005; Bright et al. 2010]. All environmental samples were stored and shipped on dry ice at -20°C to -70°C to NIOSH HELD, Morgantown, West Virginia. The samples were analyzed for the presence of pH1N1 and seasonal influenza viruses using real-time RT-PCR methodology. Additional information about our surface swab sampling is in the appendix. Figures 4–6 show some of the surfaces on which we collected swab samples.

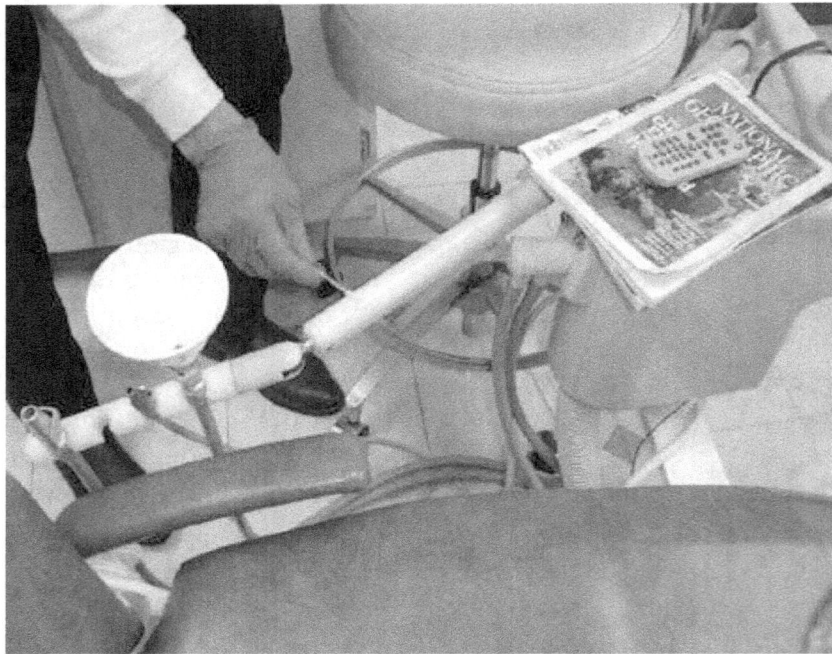

Figure 4. NIOSH investigator obtains a surface swab sample on a dental equipment support structure.

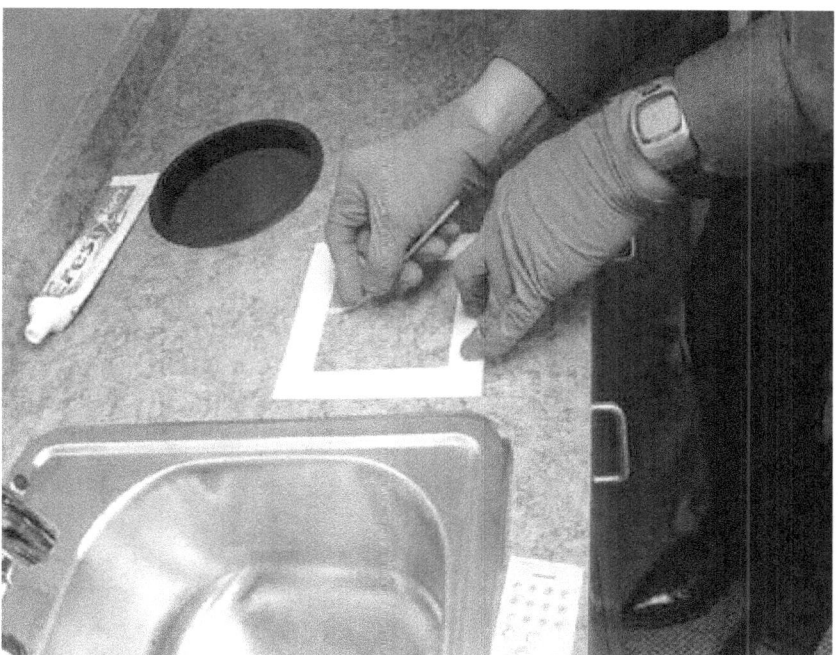

Figure 5. NIOSH investigator obtains a surface swab sample on the counter next to a sink used by patients during tooth brushing.

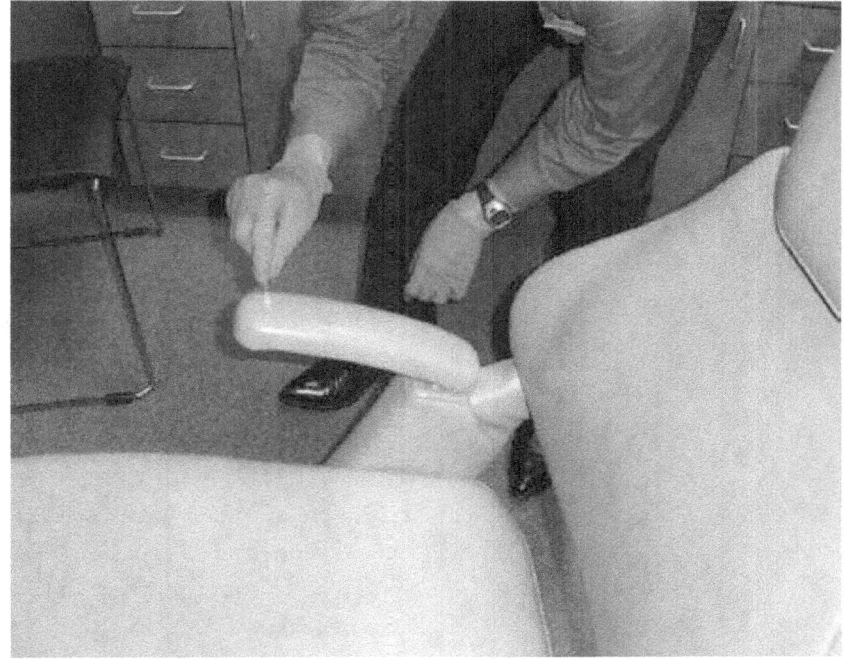

Figure 6. NIOSH investigator obtains a surface swab sample on a dental chair armrest.

We submitted spiked positive controls for seasonal influenza A to the analytic laboratory to determine if there were potential problems with field sampling or lab analysis procedures. Positive controls indistinguishable from our field samples were submitted to the lab and handled the same way as our field samples and field blanks.

We obtained additional environmental information for the patient areas using two HHPC samplers (ART Instruments, Grants Pass, Oregon). We placed HHPC units alongside two of the aerosol samplers during each day we sampled for pH1N1 and seasonal influenza. The HHPC provides a total count for particles falling into one of six size ranges: 0.3–0.5 μm, 0.5–1.0 μm, 1.0–3.0 μm, 3.0–5.0 μm, 5.0–10.0 μm, and > 10.0 μm. The HHPC results are not specific for viral particles. They identify the presence of all particles in the air in different size categories regardless of particle composition or source. The particle size cutoff for each of the HPPC six size ranges differs from the three particle size cutoffs of the bioaerosol sampler. We also measured indoor temperature and relative humidity data for the days we did environmental sampling.

## Medical Assessment

We invited all employees at both practices working on the HHE sampling dates to participate in the evaluation. We handed out a brief survey to all employee participants on each day of sampling. The survey addressed recent history of symptoms of ILI and recent influenza vaccination. Our definition for ILI was fever >100°F along with a cough and/or sore throat (http://www.cdc.gov/flu/weekly/fluactivity.htm), which was the CDC definition.

After obtaining informed consent, we obtained NP samples from each participating employee on each sampling date. The samples were analyzed at the NIOSH HELD analytical laboratory for the presence of pH1N1 and seasonal influenza viruses using real-time RT-PCR methodology. NP samples collected on February 8, 2010; February 23, 2010; and March 2, 2010, were also analyzed for RSV using the same methodology. Following each week of sampling, we informed each employee participant in writing of the results of his or her nasopharyngeal swab test and its significance.

We also developed a brief survey for patients. As part of the patient registration process, dental practice staff handed out this survey to all patients seeking dental care (or to their parents if the patients were less than 18 years of age) on the HHE sampling dates. The survey was voluntary and addressed recent history of influenza symptoms and recent influenza vaccination of the patient and any accompanying individuals. Dental practice staff collected the completed surveys and placed them in the individual patient's dental record. We then abstracted the information (without personal identifiers) from the patient's dental record. We did not have direct contact with patients during this process, and we did not collect nasopharyngeal samples from patients.

# RESULTS

## Exposure Assessment

### Dental Practice A

No pH1N1 or seasonal influenza A virus was detected using RT-PCR on the 48 air samples or 52 surface swab samples we obtained at Dental Practice A. Airborne particles within the size ranges we would have expected to find influenza viruses were present during the days we sampled, based upon the real-time HHPC data collected alongside two of our bioaerosol samplers located about 6 feet from the dental chair headrest. (Note the HHPC and two-stage bioaerosol sampler sitting on top of the half-wall at the left side of Figure 2.) Figure 7 presents an example of the HHPC total particle counts for six size fractions obtained on January 27, 2010, at Dental Practice A.

Note that the top two lines in Figure 7 present particle counts for particle sizes ($\leq$ 1μm) that are also collected in the final stage of the NIOSH bioaerosol sampler. The particle counts presented on the third and fourth lines down from the top in Figure 7 overlap with the 1–4.1 μm size particles collected by the second stage of the bioaerosol sampler. The bottom three lines plotting airborne particle size in Figure 7 correspond with the particle sizes captured in the first stage of the bioaerosol sampler, (all particles $\geq$ 4.1μm in size).

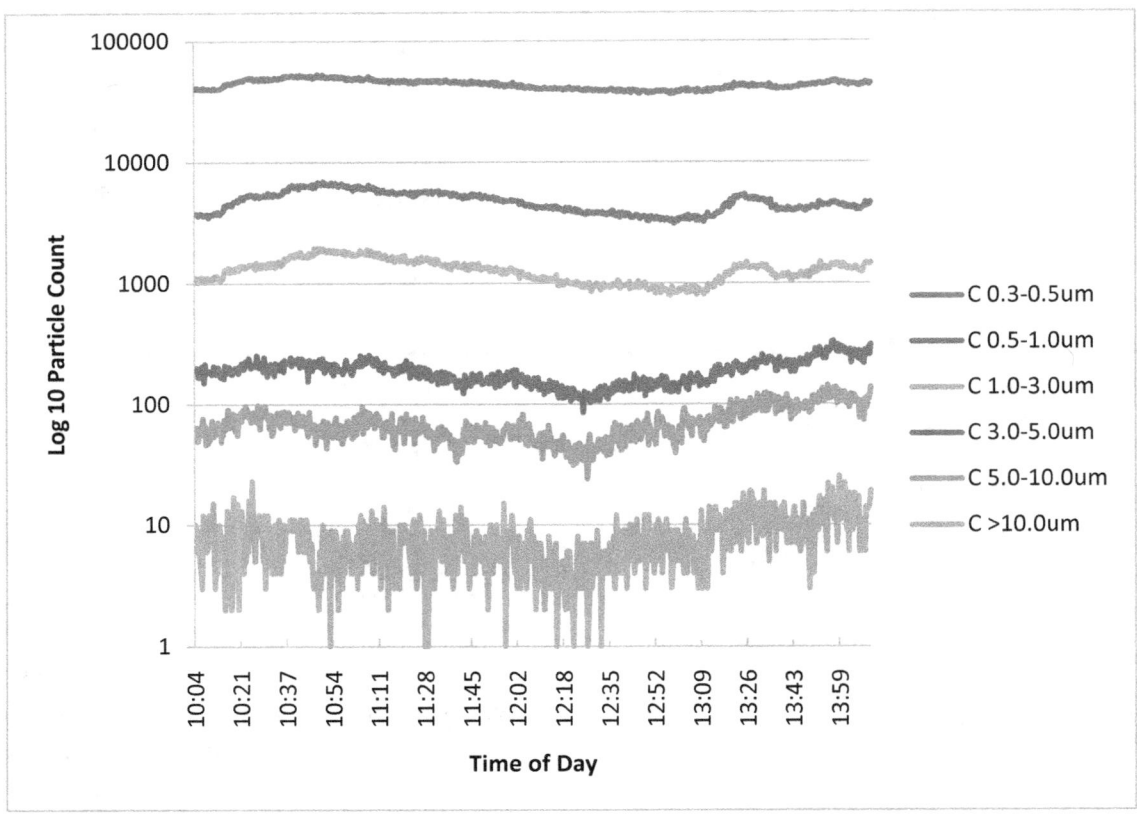

Figure 7. Plot of HHPC data of total particle count versus sample time for six airborne particle size fractions obtained January 27, 2010, Dental Practice A, room 4.

### Dental Practice B

No pH1N1 was identified in the 48 air samples collected at Dental Practice B. However, we identified seasonal influenza A on the filter stage only (≤ 1μm in size) of the bioaerosol samplers mounted on the dental exam light in rooms three, five, and six on March 2, 2010. In room three, the positive seasonal influenza A response on the bioaerosol sampler filter was subtyped as influenza H3N2. Analytical limitations prevented any further subtyping of the seasonal influenza A virus particles found on the other two positive samples. No seasonal influenza A virus was identified in the first two stages for any of these three samplers (particle sizes ≥ 4.1 μm and 1–4.1 μm). However, other airborne particles within these size ranges were identified using the HPPC located alongside two of our bioaerosol samplers (Figure 8).

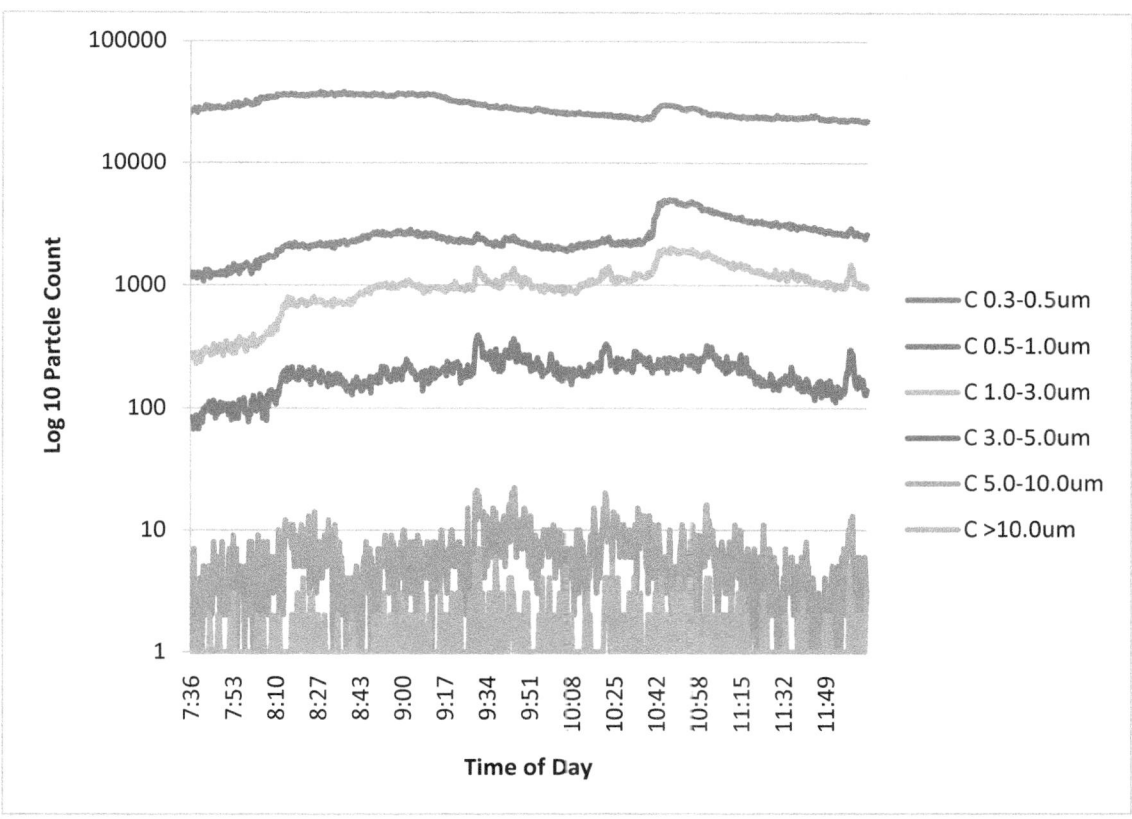

Figure 8. Plot of HHPC data of total particle count versus sample time for six airborne particle size fractions obtained March 2, 2010, Dental Practice B, on half-wall between Rooms 3 and 4. (See left side of Figure 2.)

The 54 surface samples obtained at Dental Practice B in the same rooms where air samples were collected were all negative for pH1N1 and seasonal influenza A viruses.

Samples collected on February 8, 2010; February 23, 2010; and March 2, 2010, at Dental Practice B were also analyzed for RSV. One air and one surface swab sample, both obtained in room two on March 2, 2010, were positive for RSV. RSV was detected in the first stage (≥ 4.1 μm size particles) of the aerosol sampler located on the dental exam light above the patient dental chair. The RSV positive surface swab was collected on the right armrest of the same chair. All air and surface sampling results for both dental practices are summarized in Table 1.

Table 1. Summary Sampling Results for Viruses in Airborne and Surface Swab Samples Obtained at Two Dental Practices from January 26 to March 2, 2010

| Dental Practice | Sample Type | Total No. Samples | # pH1N1 Positive | # Seasonal Influenza Positive | # RSV Positive (Practice B) |
|---|---|---|---|---|---|
| Dental Practice A | Bioaerosol size fraction: | | | | |
| | ≥ 4.1 µm | 48 | 0 | 0 | NA* |
| | 1.0–4.1 µm | 48 | 0 | 0 | NA |
| | ≤ 1 µm | 48 | 0 | 0 | NA |
| | Surface swabs | 52 | 0 | 0 | NA |
| Dental Practice B | Bioaerosol size fraction: | | | | |
| | ≥ 4.1 µm | 48 | 0 | 0 | 1 |
| | 1.0–4.1 µm | 48 | 0 | 0 | 0 |
| | ≤ 1 µm | 48 | 0 | 3 | 0 |
| | Surface swabs | 54 | 0 | 0 | 1 |
| Total samples (%) | Bioaerosol samples (air) | 96 (100%) | 0 | 3 (3%) | 1/36 (3%)† (Practice B) |
| | Surface swabs | 106 (100%) | 0 | 0 | 1/42 (2%)† (Practice B) |

*NA = RSV analyses for Dental Practice A not requested, not applicable.

†Qualitative analyses of air and wipe samples for RSV were obtained for samples collected at Dental Practice B only for the sampling dates of February 8, 2010; February 23, 2010; and March 2, 2010; resulting in the lower total number of samples evaluated for the presence of RSV.

## Medical Assessment

All employees working at both dental practices completed surveys on the sampling dates. Participation rates of employees in the NP sampling ranged from 55%–100% at Dental Practice A and ranged from 73%–100% at Dental Practice B on the sampling dates). All NP samples collected from dental practice staff at both practices were negative for influenza A viruses. All NP samples collected from employees at Dental Practice B on February 8, 2010; February 23, 2010; and March 2, 2010; were also negative for RSV.

During sampling visits on January 27, 2010; February 2, 2010; and February 24, 2010, at Dental Practice A, none of the employees, patients, or individuals accompanying patients who completed symptom surveys reported symptoms consistent with ILI in the prior 7 days. During our third sampling visit on February 17, 2010, none of the employees reported symptoms consistent with ILI. However, one of the 32 patients and one of the 8 individuals accompanying patients did report symptoms consistent with ILI. Thus, a total of 2 of 185 (1%) reported ILI symptoms on the sampling dates at Dental Practice A.

During our first sampling visit to Dental Practice B on January 26, 2010, one of the 14 employees and three of the 14 patients who completed symptom surveys reported symptoms consistent with ILI in the prior 7 days. None of the individuals accompanying patients on this date who completed symptoms surveys reported ILI symptoms. During our second sampling visit on February 8, 2010, none of the employees or individuals accompanying patients reported ILI symptoms. However, one of the 15 patients did report ILI symptoms. During our third sampling visit on February 23, 2010, none of the employees reported ILI symptoms. However, one of the 14 patients and one of the 16 individuals accompanying patients reported ILI symptoms. During our fourth sampling visit on March 2, 2010, none of the employees, patients, or individuals accompanying patients reported ILI symptoms. Thus, a total of seven of 123 (6%) individuals reported ILI symptoms on the sampling dates at Dental Practice B, the majority of whom were patients.

Self-reported vaccination rates for employees at Dental Practice A through February 24, 2010, were 8% (1 of 12 employees) for pH1N1 and 25% (3 of 12 employees) for seasonal influenza. Self-reported vaccination rates for employees at Dental Practice B through March 2, 2010 were 18% (3 of 17 employees) for pH1N1 and 18% (3 of 17 employees) for seasonal influenza (Table 2).

Self-reported vaccination rates for patients at Dental Practice A on the sampling dates were 20% (26 of 130 patients) for pH1N1 and 42% (55 of 130 patients) for seasonal influenza. Parent-reported vaccination rates for pediatric patients at Dental Practice B on the sampling dates were 64% (32 of 50 patients) for pH1N1 and 48% (24 of 50 patients) for seasonal influenza (Table 2).

Table 2. Self-reported pH1N1 and Seasonal Influenza Vaccination Rates Among Employees and Patients

| Dental Practice | Employees pH1N1 (%) | Employees Seasonal (%) | Patients pH1N1 (%) | Patients Seasonal (%) |
|---|---|---|---|---|
| A | 1/12 (8) | 3/12 (25) | 26/130 (20) | 55/130 (55) |
| B | 3/17 (18) | 3/17 (18) | 32/50 (64) | 24/50 (48) |

# Discussion

Dental employees providing direct patient care have the potential for close contact with patients during dental procedures. Additionally, employees in a dental practice may encounter patients and colleagues who could be shedding influenza virus with or without accompanying influenza symptoms. Dental employees do not perform aerosol generating procedures identified by SHEA to be "high risk" [CDC 2010b, SHEA 2009]. However, they perform procedures, such as tooth preparation with a rotary instrument or air abrasion, use of an air-water syringe or ultrasonic scaler, and air polishing, that may result in aerosolization of influenza viruses because the mouth may harbor bacteria and viruses from the nose, throat, and respiratory passages [Harrel and Molinari 2004].

Influenza infections occur through three primary modes of exposure: droplet transmission, contact transmission, and aerosol transmission. The relative contribution of these three modes of transmission is unknown and remains a subject of debate [Atkinson and Wein 2008]. The generally accepted primary mode of transmission for influenza is via droplet spread [SHEA 2009]. Previous measurement for airborne influenza virus in a hospital emergency department identified 53% of the detectable influenza virus particles within the respirable aerosol ($\leq 4.1$ μm size) fraction [Blachere et al. 2009]. An observational study of influenza virus in human exhaled breath reported that $> 99\%$ of exhaled particles were $< 5.0$ μm [Fabian et al. 2008]. Researchers evaluating the size distribution of droplets in the exhaled breath of healthy human subjects from mouth breathing, nose breathing, coughing, and talking found that the majority of particles were $\leq 1$μm [Papineni and Rosenthal 1997].

# DISCUSSION
## (CONTINUED)

The peak month for seasonal influenza cases in the Northern hemisphere from 1976–1977 through 2008–2009 has been February followed by January, March, and December [CDC 2009c]. However, the 2009–2010 influenza season did not follow this pattern. The pH1N1 influenza virus first appeared in late April 2009, with resurgence in September and October 2009. Uncertainty existed regarding whether a third resurgence would occur. We initiated our exposure assessment during the last week of January 2010 when influenza activity was below typical seasonal influenza levels; no resurgence or "third wave" of pH1N1 occurred. Because we did not find any pH1N1 and very little seasonal influenza viruses in our environmental samples, we suspended our field evaluation after completing four weeks of sampling. Figure 9 shows that the weekly percent of visits for ILI continued to decline below the Region 5 seasonal ILI baseline of 1.7% of outpatient visits [National Center for Infectious Diseases 2010]. The annual influenza season normally starts during the first full week of October. Our first week of sampling began on week 4 of the calendar year. Our last 2 weeks of sampling occurred during weeks 8 and 9. Figure 9 shows that by this time the second wave of peak pH1N1 activity was over and the likelihood of additional pH1N1 infections continued to decline.

Considering that only 3% (3 of 96) of our air samples for influenza A viruses were positive and none were positive for pH1N1, exposure of dental staff at both practices to airborne influenza A viruses during the sampling days appears to have been limited. The HHPC results indicated that even though we saw no influenza A viruses, particles in the size range where we would expect to find influenza viruses were present in both dental practices. The HHPC results indicated that even though influenza A viruses were not present, it was not because particulates within the size range which would include influenza viruses were not present in the patient rooms.

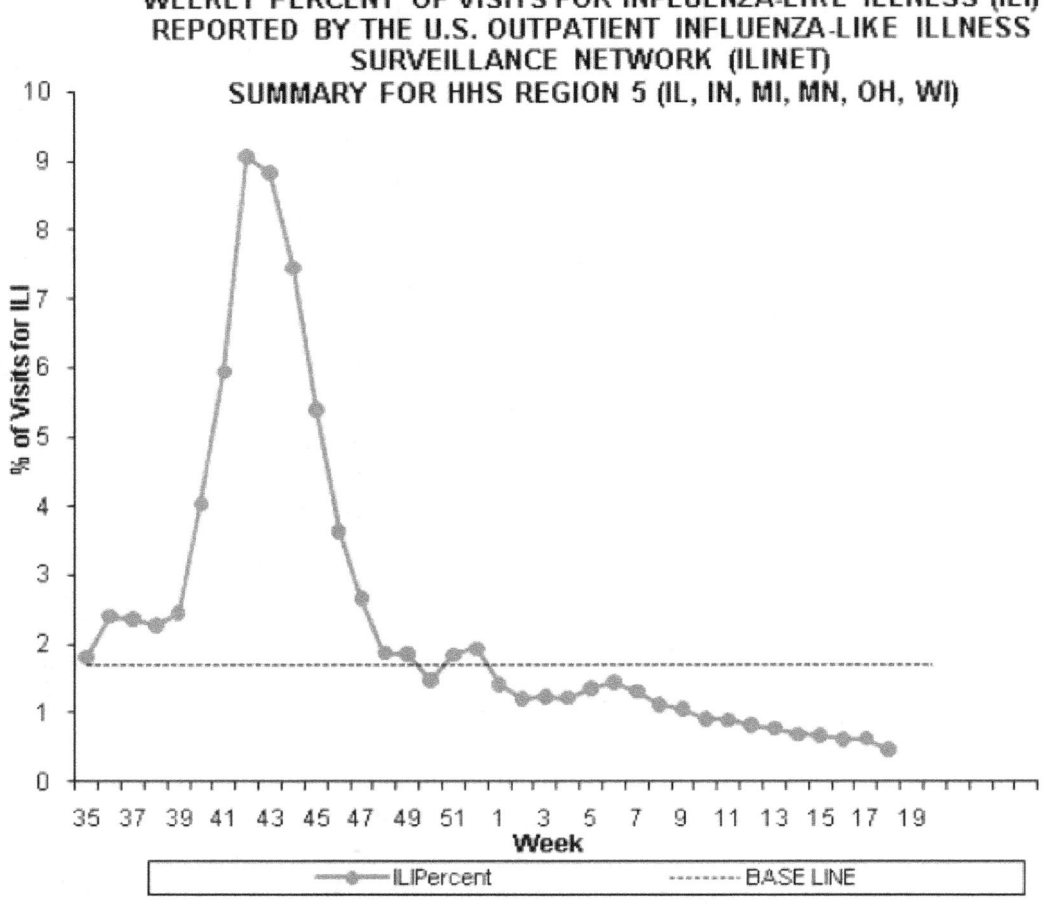

Figure 9. Region 5 weekly percent of visits for ILI for the 2009–2010 influenza season through May 8, 2010 (week 18) [National Center for Infectious Diseases 2010].

It is not surprising that we only had a few positive results for seasonal influenza virus strains in the environmental samples. During a period similar to our sampling dates (January 24– March 6, 2010), CDC reported that 99%–100% of subtyped influenza A viruses reported to CDC were pH1N1 viruses. This demonstrates the low circulating activity of non-pH1N1 influenza virus strains [CDC 2009b]. The continuing decline of ILI within the community meant that it was less likely dental staff would encounter patients, patient family members, or coworkers shedding pH1N1 or seasonal influenza viruses. Because of the low level of pH1N1 and seasonal influenza activity, we are unable to draw conclusions about general risk of exposure for dental staff during periods of higher influenza activity.

# DISCUSSION
(CONTINUED)

The absence of positive surface swab samples for influenza A viruses may be primarily due to the low number of patients reporting ILI. Additionally, the surface disinfection procedures used by dental staff between patients may have also effectively removed surface contamination by influenza A virus, if present. Direct contact surfaces in the patient rooms at both dental practices are wiped down with disinfectant spray or wipes after each patient. As mentioned earlier in this report, other investigators have identified the presence of influenza A virus on up to 50% of surfaces tested during the influenza season [Boone and Gerba 2005; Bright et al. 2010].

The negative results from our environmental samples during the first days of sampling reinforced our decision to prepare and submit (to the analyst) unidentified positive samples along with our field samples and blanks. We wanted to determine that we didn't have a problem with the handling and shipping of our completed field samples prior to their arrival at the laboratory. The analyst identified all of the positive control samples we submitted.

We observed dental staff at both practices using face shields, safety glasses, procedure masks, and disposable gloves when working with patients. Because of the low levels of exposure we found, we are unable to assess the adequacy of the personal protective equipment used by the dental staff. The three influenza A positive air samples that we did find were all associated with the smallest size fraction of airborne particulate ($\leq 1$ μm) and were all obtained at a location close to where dental staff work (immediately above the dental exam light). Procedure masks are not considered respiratory protection and are not designed to filter this size of particulate [Brosseau et al. 1997]. CDC recommended the use of NIOSH-certified respiratory protection that was at least as protective as a fit-tested disposable N95 respirator for healthcare personnel who were in close contact with patients with suspected or confirmed pH1N1. This recommendation applied uniquely to the special circumstances of the pH1N1 pandemic during the fall and winter of 2009–2010 [CDC 2010c]. Facemasks that have been cleared for marketing by the U.S. Food and Drug Administration have been tested for their ability to resist blood and body fluids, and generally provide a physical barrier to droplets that are expelled directly at the user. Although they do not efficiently filter small particles from the air and they allow leakage around the mask, they are a barrier to splashes, droplet sprays, and autoinoculation of influenza virus from the hands to the nose and mouth.

All NP samples collected from employees at both dental practices on all sampling dates were negative for influenza A viruses. These results were anticipated, as none of the employees at Dental Practice A reported ILI symptoms, and only one employee at Dental Practice B reported ILI symptoms on just one sampling date. Our survey results demonstrate the low prevalence of ILI symptoms, 1% at Dental Practice A and 4% at Dental Practice B, among employees and patients during this 5-week period. This is consistent with the CDC reports at the time, which documented low influenza and ILI activity. In addition, these results suggest that dental staff did not come to work when ill and very few patients visited the dental practice when ill on the sampling dates.

pH1N1 vaccination rates for employees were 8% for Dental Practice A and 18% for Dental Practice B. Though CDC's ACIP recommended that healthcare personnel be among the target groups to receive the pH1N1 vaccine first [CDC 2009e], vaccination rates among these dental employees were suboptimal. These rates are also well below the estimated pH1N1 vaccination rate among employees in ambulatory, outpatient, and dental practices nationwide as of mid-January, which was 39% [CDC 2010d].

Seasonal influenza vaccination rates for employees were 25% for Dental Practice A and 18% for Dental Practice B. CDC's ACIP has had longstanding recommendations that target groups for seasonal influenza vaccination include all healthcare personnel [CDC 2009a]. Despite this, seasonal influenza vaccination rates among the dental employees were also suboptimal. These rates are also well below the estimated seasonal influenza vaccination rate of 64% among employees in ambulatory, outpatient, and dental practices nationwide as of mid-January [CDC 2010d].

The self-reported pH1N1 vaccination rate for Dental Practice A patients, consisting of mostly adults, was 20%. This rate was similar to the estimated pH1N1 vaccination rate among adults in the state of Ohio, which was 18% as of the end of January 2010 [CDC 2010e]. The parent-reported pH1N1 vaccination rate for patients (all children) at Dental Practice B was 67%. This is higher than the estimated pH1N1 vaccination rate among children in the state of Ohio, which was 34% as of the end of January 2010 [CDC 2010e]. Our findings are consistent with CDC's findings that vaccination coverage was higher among children than adults, largely thought to be due to school-based vaccination programs. The higher than expected pH1N1 vaccination rates among Dental Practice A and

B patients may have been one of the factors that contributed to the fact that pH1N1 virus was not detected in the air and surface sampling.

The self-reported seasonal influenza vaccination rate for Dental Practice A patients was 42%. This rate was similar to the estimated seasonal influenza vaccination rate among adults in the state of Ohio, which was 41% as of the end of January, 2010 [CDC 2010f]. The parent-reported rate for Dental Practice B patients was 48%. This is higher than the estimated seasonal influenza vaccination rate among children in the state of Ohio, which was 39% as of the end of January, 2010 [CDC 2010f]. These relatively high rates of seasonal influenza vaccination may have been one of the factors that contributed to the fact that seasonal influenza virus was not detected in the air or environmental samples.

Our evaluation was subject to some limitations. The continuing decline in influenza activity below seasonal levels may have contributed to the absence of pH1N1 and seasonal influenza during our exposure assessment. The identification of influenza and respiratory viruses collected using the NIOSH two-stage bioaerosol sampler does not provide any indication of the collected virus' viability or infectivity. (Note that determining the viability of collected airborne viruses was not an objective of this evaluation.)

The absence of influenza viruses in the work environment we evaluated prevented looking at near versus distant samplers' ability to collect influenza viruses. Our results do not provide any insight into whether exposure is limited to close proximity to the potential source (patient) or if the virus may also be airborne at a distance at or beyond 6 feet. Air sampler spacing distances and location were limited by room and equipment configurations and do not represent individual dental staff breathing zone exposures.

HHPC data does not correlate exactly with the size fractions collected by the two-stage bioaerosol sampler and it does not provide any information on the composition or source of particulates making up the six different size fractions reported by the HPPC for samples collected at both dental practices.

We did not identify the primary dental procedures performed for each patient within a room during the sampling period. Our results cannot provide information about the potential for exposure to influenza virus from the patients under current working conditions in the dental practices evaluated.

# DISCUSSION (CONTINUED)

We did not achieve 100% participation in the collection of nasopharyngeal samples among employees at both practices during all sampling dates. However, 100% of employees working on those dates did complete surveys, and none of the employees who declined to provide a nasopharyngeal sample reported ILI symptoms in the previous seven days.

Also, we were informed that some parents of patients in Dental Practice B declined to complete the surveys passed out by dental practice staff upon registration. This limited our potential to detect the source of non-pH1N1 virus found in air samples at Dental Practice B on March 2, 2010, and the source of RSV found in swab samples on the same date. It should be noted that the survey asked employees and patients about symptoms specific for ILI and did not include some of the symptoms of RSV infection.

Our vaccination rates were based on self and parents reports and may have been subject to recall bias. Vaccination was not validated by medical records, and persons may have confused receipt of the pH1N1 and seasonal influenza vaccinations.

# CONCLUSIONS

Because of low incidence of ILI among dental staff, patients, and within the community, we could not successfully evaluate the potential for exposure of dental staff to pH1N1 or seasonal influenza. We found no pH1N1 in any of the air samples and we only found influenza A in three samples at Dental Practice B on one day. Neither dental staff nor patients were coming in with ILI symptoms. Immunization rates among dental staff for both pH1N1 and seasonal influenza were below the rates reported for the 2009–2010 influenza season among health care workers. They were also lower than the influenza immunization rates reported by their patients. Both dental practices followed standard precautions regarding infection control procedures and use of PPE in dental practices.

# RECOMMENDATIONS

Based on our findings, we recommend the actions listed below to create a more healthful workplace. We encourage the dental practices to discuss the recommendations in this report with all employees and jointly develop an action plan. Those involved in the work can best set priorities and assess the feasibility of our recommendations for their dental practices. Our recommendations are based on the occupational safety and health hierarchy of controls approach. This approach groups actions by their likely effectiveness in reducing or removing hazards. In most cases, the preferred approach is to eliminate hazardous materials or processes and install engineering controls to reduce exposure or shield employees. Until such controls are in place, or if they are not effective or feasible, administrative measures and/or personal protective equipment may be needed.

## Elimination and Substitution

Eliminating the potential source of exposure is a highly effective means for reducing hazards and ranks highest in the hierarchy of controls.

1. Develop procedures for monitoring and managing employees who are ill and absent.

    a. Encourage employees to self-assess for ILI symptoms and report symptoms to their supervisor.

    b. Exclude employees with ILI symptoms from work according to the most recent CDC guidance, which can be found on the CDC website at http://www.cdc.gov/flu/professionals/infectioncontrol/healthcaresettings.htm.

2. Consider developing mechanisms to screen patients for ILI symptoms prior to their visits, such as through the appointment reminder system. Consider requesting symptomatic patients to postpone elective visits and procedures until 24 hours after they are free of fever, especially in times of high influenza activity.

## Administrative Controls

Administrative controls are management-dictated work practices and policies to reduce or prevent exposures to workplace hazards. The effectiveness of administrative changes in work practices for controlling workplace hazards is dependent on management commitment and employee acceptance. Regular monitoring and reinforcement is necessary to ensure that control policies and procedures are not circumvented in the name of convenience or production.

1. Encourage all employees to receive the annual seasonal influenza vaccine. The 2010–2011 seasonal influenza vaccine will protect against pH1N1 and two other influenza viruses. Consider instituting an employer requirement of influenza vaccine as part of a comprehensive influenza infection control strategy. This has been associated with higher rates of seasonal influenza vaccination compared with rates among health care providers whose employers neither required nor recommended seasonal influenza vaccination [CDC 2010g]. The WHO continues to encourage vaccination as an important preventive measure to reduce morbidity and mortality caused by influenza viruses during the post-pandemic period of pH1N1 announced August 10, 2010 [World Health Organization 2010]. Explore the feasibility of offering seasonal influenza vaccination to employees at the worksite [CDC 2006].

2. Identify patients with ILI by symptom screen and/or temperature check at check-in and reschedule those presenting for non-urgent care. If evaluating for urgent care, offer the patient a facemask to wear prior to dental procedures and separate ill patients from others whenever possible.

## Personal Protective Equipment

PPE use in dental offices is a part of routine general infection control practices [CDC 2010h]. However, PPE use for influenza transmission prevention is the least effective means for controlling employee exposure and should not be relied upon as the sole method for limiting employee exposures. Proper use of PPE requires a comprehensive program, and calls for a high level of employee involvement and commitment to be effective. The latest CDC PPE recommendations for healthcare personnel who are in close contact with patients with confirmed or suspected influenza can be found at http://www.cdc.gov/flu/professionals/infectioncontrol/healthcaresettings.htm.

# REFERENCES

Atkinson MP, Wein LM [2008]. Quantifying the routes of transmission for pandemic influenza. Bull Math Biol 70(3):820–867.

Blachere FM, Lindsley WG, Pearce TA, Anderson SE, Fisher M, Khakoo R, Meade BJ, Lander O, Davis S, Thewlis RE, Celik I, Chen BT, Beezhold DH [2009]. Measurement of airborne influenza virus in a hospital emergency department. Clin Infect Dis 48(15):438–440.

Boone SA, Gerba CP [2005]. The Occurence of Influenza A Virus on Household and Day Care Center Fomites. J Infect 51(2):103–109.

Bright KR, Boone SA, Gerba CP [2010]. Occurrence of bacteria and viruses on elementary classroom surfaces and the potential role of classroom hygiene in the spread of infectious diseases. Journal of School Nursing 26(1):33–41.

Brosseau LM, McCullough NV, Vesley D [1997]. Mycobacterial aerosol collection efficiency of respirator and surgical mask filters under varying conditions of flow and humidity. Applied Occup Environ Hyg 12(6):435–445.

CDC [2006]. Influenza Vaccination of Health-Care Personnel. Recommendations of the Healthcare Infection Control Practices Advisory Committee (HICPAC) and the Advisory Committee on Immunization Practices (ACIP). MMWR 55(RR02);1–16.

CDC [2009a]. 2009 H1N1 Flu ("Swine Flu") and You. [http://www.cdc.gov/H1N1flu/qa.htm]. Date accessed: December 2010.

CDC [2009b]. 2009 H1N1 Vaccination Recommendations. [http://www.cdc.gov/h1n1flu/vaccination/acip.html]. Date accessed: December 2010.

CDC [2009c]. Prevention and control of sesonal influenza with vaccines: Recommendation of the Advisory Committee on Immunization Practices (ACIP). MMWR 58(RR-8):1–52.

CDC [2009d]. Seasonal influenza (flu) - The flu season. [http://www.cdc.gov/flu/about/season/flu-season.htm] Date accessed: December 2010.

## REFERENCES
### (CONTINUED)

CDC [2009e]. 2009 H1N1 early outbreak and disease characteristics. Atlanta, GA:U.S. Department of Health and Human Services, CDC. [http://www.cdc.gov/h1n1flu/surveillanceqa.htm]. Date accessed: September 2010.

CDC [2010a]. Interim guidance on infection control measures for 2009 H1N1 influenza in healthcare settings, including protection of healthcare personnel. [http://www.cdc.gov/h1n1flu/guidelines_infection_control.htm]. Date accessed: December 2010.

CDC [2010b]. Seasonal influenza (flu): Guidelines and recommendations: Prevention strategies for seasonal influenza in health care settings. [http://www.cdc.gov/flu/professionals/infectioncontrol/healthcaresettings.htm]. Date accessed: December 2010.

CDC [2010c]. Interim results: influenza A (H1N1) 2009 monovalent and seasonal influenza vaccination coverage among health-care personnel - United States, August 2009 – January 2010. MMWR 59(12):357–362.

CDC [2010d]. Interim results: state-specific influenza A (H1N1) 2009 monovalent vaccination coverage - United States, October 2009 – January 2010. MMWR 59(12):363–368.

CDC [2010e]; Interim Results: State-Specific Seasonal Influenza Vaccination Coverage ~ United States, August 2009–January 2010. MMWR 59(16);477–484.

CDC [2010f]. Past Weekly Surveillance Reports. [http://www.cdc.gov/flu/weekly/pastreports htm]. Date accessed: December 2010.

CDC [2010g]. Updated CDC estimates of 2009 H1N1 influenza cases, hospitalizations and deaths in the United States, April 2009 – April 10, 2010 [http://www.cdc.gov/h1n1flu/estimates_2009_h1n1.htm]. Date accessed: December 2010.

CDC [2010h]. Infection control in dental settings: Personal protective equipment (Masks, protective eyewear, protective apparel, gloves). [http://www.cdc.gov/oralhealth/infectioncontrol/faq/protective_equipment.htm]. Date accessed: December 2010.

Fabian P, McDevitt JJ, DeHaan WH, Fung ROP, Cowling BJ, Chan KH, Leung GM, Milton DK [2008]. Influenza virus in

# REFERENCES
## (CONTINUED)

human exhaled breath: An observational study. PLoS ONE[serial online]3(7):e2691.

Harrel SK, Molinari J [2004]. Aerosols and splatter in dentistry: a brief review of the literature and infection control implications. The Journal of the American Dental Association 135(4):429–437.

Lindsley WG, Schmechel D, Chen BT [2006]. A two-stage cyclone using microcentrifuge tubes for personal bioaerosol sampling. J Environ Monit 8(11):1136–1142.

Lindsley WG, Blachere FM, Davis KA, Pearce TA, Fisher MA, Khakoo R, Davis SM, Rogers ME, Thewlis RE, Posada JA, Redrow JB, Celik IB, Chen BT, Beezhold DH [2010]. Distribution of airborne influenza virus and respiratory syncytial virus in an urgent care medical clinic. Clin Infect Dis 5(6):693–698.

National Center for Infectious Diseases [2010]. Weekly percentage of visits for influenza-like illness (ILI) reported by the U.S. outpatient influenza-like illness surveillance network (ILINET). [http://www.cdc.gov/flu/weekly/regions2009-2010/senreg5.html]. Date accessed: May 2010.

Papineni RS, Rosenthal FS [1997]. The Size and Distribution of Droplets in the Exhaled Breath of Healthy Human Subjects. J Aerosol Med 10(2):105–116.

SHEA [2009]. SHEA position statement: Interim guidance on infection control precautions for novel swine-origin influenza A H1N1 in healthcare facilities. Arlington, VA: The Society for Healthcare Epidemiology of America.

Siegel JD, Rhinehart E, Jackson M, Chiarello L, Healthcare Infection Control Practices Advisory Committee [2007]. 2007 Guideline for isolation precautions: Preventing transmission of infectious agents in healthcare settings. Atlanta, GA: Centers for Disease Control and Prevention, pp 17–18.

World Health Organization [2010]. WHO recommendations for the post-pandemic period: Pandemic (H1N1) 2009 briefing note 23. [http://www.who.int/csr/disease/swineflu/notes/briefing_20100810/en/index.html]. Date accessed: December 2010.

# APPENDIX: METHODS

## Environmental Sampling

### *Aerosol Sampling*

Air samples to evaluate the presence of pH1N1 and seasonal influenza viruses/viral fragments were collected using two-stage cyclone bioaerosol samplers. These samplers collect size segregated airborne particles in two standard centrifuge tubes (15 and 1.5 mL tubes, Becton Dickinson, Franklin Lakes, New Jersey) and on a PFTE filter (SKC, Inc., Eighty Four, Pennsylvania) (Figure 10) [Lindsley et al. 2006]. Aerosol samples were collected once a week at each dental facility for 4 weeks (a total of 8 sample collection days). Samples were collected for approximately 4–5 hours on each sample collection day. Sampling duration was limited to this shorter time period rather than a full work shift due to a reported decline in virus collection that occurs during longer sample periods. Air samples started with the first appointments of the day and ran continuously until 4–5 hours of time elapsed. For each day of sampling, we collected 12 air samples (96 total samples). We selected the sampling dates in consultation with the dental practices based on expected patient load, with preference given to busier days.

We located the sampling pump with the aerosol sampler on the structural support arm immediately above the dental exam light. This placed the sampler within approximately 3 feet of the patient chair. These samples acted as surrogates for personal samples. We collected an additional area sample in dental patient rooms where we had placed a sampler above the dental exam light. The selection of patient rooms targeted those rooms scheduled with a full patient load on the day of sampling. Depending on the room dimensions, configuration, and work activities, area samples were collected at a distance of 6 feet or more from the typical patient location. When room configurations allowed it, area samplers were mounted on tripods at a height of approximately 5 feet from the floor to represent standing height. Alternatively, we placed samplers on top of shelves or cabinets. In addition to samples collected in patient rooms, area samples were obtained near the patient check in location.

All air sampling pumps (SKC Aircheck XR5000, Eighty Four, Pennsylvania) were calibrated using a volumetric flow calibrator (TSI Model 4146D, Shoreview, Minnesota) to operate at a flow rate of 3.5 Lpm. At a flow rate of 3.5 Lpm, the first centrifuge tube (T1) collects particles $\geq 4.1$ µm (GSD 1.51), the second tube (T2) collects 1.0 to 4.1 µm particles (GSD 1.59) and the filter collects particles $\leq 1$ µm. At 3.5 Lpm, the sampler conforms to the ACGIH/ISO criteria for respirable particle sampling [ISO 1995]. In addition to bioaerosol samples, characterization of total particle sizes in two patient rooms was performed using an optical particle counter (ART Instruments, Inc., HHPC-6, Grants Pass, Oregon). The particle counters were placed adjacent to an area bioaerosol sampler during data collection (See Figure 2 in the report text).

The arrows show the direction of air flow through the sampler. Air is drawn through the sampler using a small portable vacuum pump. Air flows into the 15 mL first stage centrifuge tube (T1) and swirls in a cyclonic motion. Particles larger than 4.1 µm are thrown against the wall of the tube by centrifugal force, where they stick. The air and remaining particles exit the first stage, flow around a bend, and enter the 1 5 mL second stage centrifugal tube (T2). Since the second stage inlet and collection tube diameter are smaller than the first, air flow is accelerated and higher centrifugal forces are generated. Particles in the size range 1.0 to 4.1 µm are captured on the wall of the second tube. Finally, the air flows out of the second stage and passes through a 37 millimeter PTFE filter with 2.0 µm pore size (housed in a black

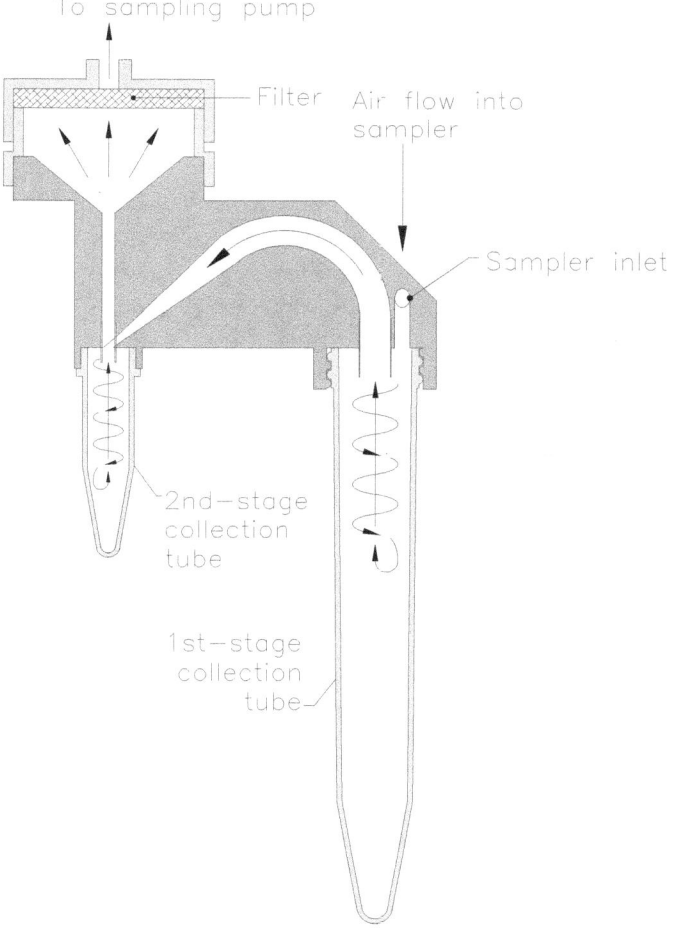

Figure 10. Schematic of the NIOSH two-stage cyclone aerosol sampler.

polypropylene conductive cassette), which captures particles smaller than 1.0 μm. The first stage has a 3 mm ID inlet, a 6.1 mm ID outlet and a 6 mm vortex finder length. The second stage has a 1.3 mm ID inlet, 3 mm vortex finder length and a 2.5 mm ID outlet. The first and second stage inlets are at a 40° angle from the horizontal. The sampler is a modified version of that described previously [Lindsley et al. 2006].

The two direct-reading, real-time instruments provided a qualitative assessment characterizing total airborne particulate levels in the dental practices across the size fraction of particles collected by the two-stage cyclone aerosol samplers. The HHPC-6 hand-held particle counter (ART Instruments, Grants Pass, Oregon) determined the airborne particle counts based on optical counting principles using laser light scattering. This instrument measured the total number of particles per liter (particles/L) of air across six specific size cut points: 0.3–0.5 μm, 0 5–1.0 μm, 1.0–3.0 μm, 3.0–5.0 μm, 5.0–10.0 μm, and > 10.0 μm [Art Instruments, Inc. 2002]. Compared to the two-stage cyclone aerosol sampler, the first two size bins (smallest particle size ranges) of the HHPC identified the total particulate count for all particulate per liter of air sampled (viral and non-viral) that could be captured on the filter (Figure 10.) of the two-stage cyclone aerosol sampler. Particles counted by the HHPC for 1.0–3.0 μm and 3.0–5.0 μm size fractions would be collected on the second stage collection tube of the two-stage cyclone aerosol sampler. HHPC counts for 3.0–5.0 μm, 5.0–10.0 μm, and > 10.0 μm airborne particles reflect the particle sizes that could be collected by the first stage of the two-stage cyclone aerosol sampler. The HHPC counts all particles in the specified size ranges regardless of composition or source that are present in each 1 liter air sample. The HHPC was set to collect three samples per minute. The HHPCs were operated during the same time period that the two-stage cyclone aerosol samples were run to collect influenza virus. The two HHPCs were located adjacent to two separate two-stage cyclone aerosol samplers (See Figure 2). While the particulate size fractions collected by the HHPC did not align exactly with those of the two-stage cyclone aerosol sampler they provided a qualitative indication of the total number of particles present in the different size ranges from which the two-stage cyclone aerosol samplers were sampling for pH1N1 and seasonal influenza virus particles.

Air samples were transported back to the NIOSH laboratory upon completion of sampling. We added 0.6 mL of lysis binding solution to the 15 and 1.5 mL centrifuge tubes from the samplers. The filters were transferred into a new 15 mL centrifuge tube and 0.5 mL of lysis binding solution added. All tubes were vortexed to distribute lysis binding solution throughout the sampling medium. These samples were also stored at -20°C and shipped on dry ice along with the surface samples to the NIOSH HELD analytical laboratory.

## Surface Sampling

We did surface sampling of common high-contact non-porous surfaces to identify the presence of pH1N1 and seasonal influenza virus. Samples were collected from some or all of the following surfaces on each day of air sampling: patient check-in/check-out countertop, doorknobs, patient room countertops, arms of patient chairs, handle of reusable dental tools (before cleaning), computer keyboard and mouse, and sink faucet handles. These samples were obtained in the same rooms where the air samples were collected. Surface samples were collected by swabbing the surfaces with sterile nylon flocked swabs (Copan Diagnostics, Corona, California) moistened with sterile phosphate buffered saline (Invitrogen, Aukland, New Zealand). For large flat surfaces a 10 cm x 10 cm template was used to collect a 100 cm2 surface area sample. For non-flat surfaces, 100 cm2 was estimated or the entire surface sampled (e.g., doorknob, dental tool handles, sink faucet handles) and the area estimated based on surface dimensions.

Immediately following collection, surface samples were placed into a 15 mL centrifuge tube (Becton Dickinson, Franklin Lakes, New Jersey) containing 0.5 mL of lysis binding solution (Ambion Diagnostics/ Applied Biosystems, Austin, Texas). Samples were stored at -20°C, then shipped on dry ice to the NIOSH HELD analytical laboratory.

## Nasopharyngeal Sampling

For NP sampling, a flexible flocked swab with a nylon tip (Copan Diagnostics, Inc., Murrieta, California) was inserted through each participant's nose into the nasopharynx until resistance was encountered. The swab was rubbed gently and rolled for several seconds to absorb secretions before removing. Samples from both nostrils were collected using the same swab. The swab was then immediately placed into a sterile vial containing 0.5 mL of lysis/binding solution concentrate. The swab stick was cut off to permit tightening of the cap. The NP samples were stored and shipped at -20°C to -70°C to the NIOSH HELD analytical laboratory.

## Laboratory Analysis

### Viral RNA Extraction

Immediately following collection, stages T1 and T2 aerosol samples were suspended in 500 µl of lysis binding solution concentrate (Ambion, Austin, Texas). Back-up filters were transferred to 50 mL polypropylene conical tubes (Becton Dickinson Labware, Franklin Lakes, New Jersey) containing 500 µl of the lysis binding solution concentrate. Nasopharyngeal swabs were placed in 15 mL polypropylene conical tubes (Becton Dickinson Labware, Franklin Lakes, New Jersey) containing 500 µl of the lysis binding solution concentrate. All aerosol and swab samples were stored at -20°C. Upon thawing, to enhance RNA extraction, each sample was spiked with carrier RNA (Ambion, Austin, Texas). Likewise, random samples were spiked with XenoRNA (Applied Biosystems, Austin, Texas), a qPCR internal control. Samples were subsequently transferred to designated wells in MagMax Express Microtiter 96-Deep Well Plates (Applied Biosystems, Austin, Texas). To complete the Lysis/Binding Solution preparation, 500 µl of isopropanol was added to each sample well. Total RNA was extracted from all samples using Applied Biosystems MagMaxTM Express-96, an automated Nucleic Acid Extractor, in conjunction with the MagMAXTM -96 Viral RNA Isolation Kit (Ambion, Austin, Texas). Following isolation, RNA was immediately transcribed into cDNA.

### cDNA Transcription

Complimentary DNA (cDNA) was generated by reverse transcription of the isolated RNA with use of the High Capacity RNA to cDNA Master Mix (Applied Biosystems). Samples were transcribed in an Eppendorf Mastercycler ep under the following conditions: 25°C for 5 minutes, 42°C for 30 minutes and 85°C for 5 minutes. All samples were stored at -20°C until qPCR analysis.

### qPCR Analysis

For real-time detection of seasonal influenza A and novel H1N1 influenza, primers and probes from the CDC Swine Influenza Virus Real-Time RT-PCR Detection Panel (CDC REF. # FLUSW01, Lot # 904303) were used. Briefly, 20 µl of TaqMan Fast Universal Master Mix (Applied Biosystems, Austin, Texas) containing either influenza A or novel H1N1 specific primers and probes at a final concentration of 0.8 µM and 0.2 µM, respectively, was added to 5 µl of sample cDNA. Reactions were performed and analyzed in the Applied Biosystems 7500 Fast Real-Time PCR System under the following cycling conditions: 95°C for 20 seconds followed by 50 cycles at 95°C for 15 seconds and 55°C for 30 seconds.

To determine the relative genome copy from seasonal influenza A-positive aerosol samples, a standard curve was generated from 10-fold serial dilutions of a plasmid-encoded influenza M1 matrix gene and analyzed concurrently with all qPCR reactions. A negative control without template was also included in all RT–PCR reactions. All reactions were run in duplicate.

Comparable to the analysis of influenza, real-time detection of RSV-positive aerosol samples was performed and analyzed in the Applied Biosystems 7500 Fast Real-Time PCR System using the following matrix specific primers and probe: Forward 5' GGA AAC ATA CGT GAA CAA GCT TCA 3', Reverse 5' CAT CGT CTT TTT CTA AGA CAT TGT ATT GA 3', Probe 6FAM- TGT GTA TGT GGA GCC TT-MGBNFQ (Applied Biosystems, Austin, Texas).

To ensure that RT-PCR inhibitors were not present, real-time PCR detection of the Xeno RNA internal control was performed separately using the Xeno RNA Control TaqMan Gene Expression Assay from the TaqMan Cells to Ct Control Kit (Applied Biosystems, Austin, Texas). Cycling conditions were as follows: 95°C for 20 seconds followed by 40 cycles at 95°C 3 seconds and 60°C for 30 seconds.

## Positive Controls

The use of positive controls for the laboratory analyses confirmed that we would see pH1N1 seasonal influenza viruses in our samples if they were present. The high specificity of PCR methods for detecting pre-selected biological agents, in this case seasonal influenza A and pH1N1, allowed us to look for the virus of interest in the presence of other particulates. The seasonal qPCR assay (which selects for Matrix gene, segment 7 in the influenza A viruses) detects all influenza A strains. All samples were analyzed first using the qPCR assay for the presence of influenza A virus strains. Positive influenza A virus samples were further sub typed for seasonal and novel H1N1 (pH1N1) influenza viruses using an H1 and H3 sub typing qPCR assay. Tests for RSV on samples from Dental Practice B did identify this common respiratory virus encountered with children and often co-circulating with influenza viruses. Positive control samples prepared and handled the same as the field samples and blank came back identifying the presence of seasonal influenza. All field blanks for air and swab samples were negative for pH1N1 and seasonal influenza. Additionally, all field blanks (swab and air sample) for Dental Practice B were negative for RSV.

# References

ART Instruments, Inc. [2002]. Hand held particle counter (HHPC-6) User manual. Grants Pass, Oregon.

ISO [1995]. Air quality - Particle size fraction definitions for health-related sampling. Geneva, Switzerland: International Organization for Standardization, p. 9.

Lindsley WG, Schmechel D, Chen BT [2006]. A two-stage cyclone using microcentrifuge tubes for personal bioaerosol sampling. J Environ Monit 8(11):1136–1142.

# ACKNOWLEDGMENTS AND AVAILABILITY OF REPORT

The Hazard Evaluations and Technical Assistance Branch (HETAB) of the National Institute for Occupational Safety and Health (NIOSH) conducts field investigations of possible health hazards in the workplace. These investigations are conducted under the authority of Section 20(a)(6) of the Occupational Safety and Health Act of 1970, 29 U S.C. 669(a)(6) which authorizes the Secretary of Health and Human Services, following a written request from any employer or authorized representative of employees, to determine whether any substance normally found in the place of employment has potentially toxic effects in such concentrations as used or found. HETAB also provides, upon request, technical and consultative assistance to federal, state, and local agencies; labor; industry; and other groups or individuals to control occupational health hazards and to prevent related trauma and disease.

The findings and conclusions in this report are those of the authors and do not necessarily represent the views of NIOSH. Mention of any company or product does not constitute endorsement by NIOSH. In addition, citations to websites external to NIOSH do not constitute NIOSH endorsement of the sponsoring organizations or their programs or products. Furthermore, NIOSH is not responsible for the content of these websites. All Web addresses referenced in this document were accessible as of the publication date.

This report was prepared by Steven H. Ahrenholz, Scott E. Brueck, and Marie A. de Perio of HETAB, Division of Surveillance, Hazard Evaluations and Field Studies, and Francoise Blachere and William G. Lindsley of the Health Effects Laboratory Division (HELD). Analytical support was provided by Francoise Blachere and Don Beezhold, HELD. Health communication assistance was provided by Stefanie Evans. Editorial assistance was provided by Ellen Galloway. Desktop publishing was performed by Robin Smith.

Copies of this report have been sent to employee and management representatives at both dental practices, the state health department, and the Occupational Safety and Health Administration Regional Office. This report is not copyrighted and may be freely reproduced. The report may be viewed and printed at www.cdc.gov/niosh/hhe/. Copies may be purchased from the National Technical Information Service at 5825 Port Royal Road, Springfield, Virginia 22161.

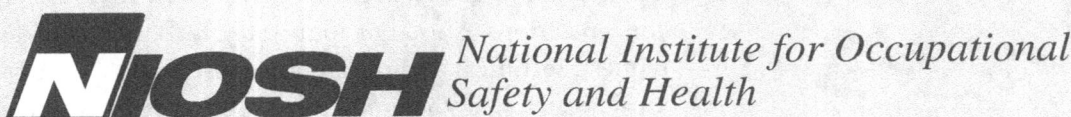
National Institute for Occupational Safety and Health

# Delivering on the Nation's promise: Safety and health at work for all people through research and prevention.

To receive NIOSH documents or information about occupational safety and health topics, contact NIOSH at:

**1-800-CDC-INFO** (1-800-232-4636)

TTY: 1-888-232-6348

E-mail: cdcinfo@cdc.gov

or visit the NIOSH web site at: **www.cdc.gov/niosh.**

For a monthly update on news at NIOSH, subscribe to NIOSH eNews by visiting **www.cdc.gov/niosh/eNews.**

SAFER • HEALTHIER • PEOPLE™

www.ingramcontent.com/pod-product-compliance
Lightning Source LLC
Chambersburg PA
CBHW080927290526
45795CB00007BA/2677